THE ULTIMATE CROCK POT SLOW COOKER RECIPES 2021

DELICIOUS CROCK POT RECIPES EASY TO MAKE

JIM CURTIS

Copyright © 2021

Edited by: Jim Curtis

Cover by: Jim Curtis

All rights reserved. No part of this publication may be reproduced, stored in a retrieval system, or transmitted in any form or by any means, electronic, mechanical, recording or otherwise, without the prior written permission of the author.

2021

Table of Contents

Cranberry Sauce 15

Ingredients 15

Preparation 15

Fig Apple Butter 16

Ingredients 16

Preparation 16

Fruit and Berry Cobbler 17

Ingredients 17

Preparation 17

Greek Yogurt 19

Ingredients 19

Preparation 19

Paleo Slow Cooker Ketchup 21

Ingredients 21

Preparation 21

Pumpkin Butter 23

Ingredients 23

Preparation 23

Paleo Pumpkin Pie Pudding 24

Ingredients 24

Preparation 24

Spiced Hot Apple Cidar 25

Ingredients 25

Preparation 25

Strawberry Applesauce 26

Ingredients 26

Preparation 26

Vanilla Bean Honeycrisp Applesauce 27

Ingredients 27

Preparation 27

Yogurt, Kid-Made! 28

Ingredients 28

Preparation 28

Cinnamon Apple Oatmeal 29

Ingredients 29

Preparation 29

Banana Bread Quinoa 30

Ingredients 30

Preparation 30

Vegetable Breakfast Burritos 31

Ingredients 31

Preparation 31

Greek Yogurt 32

Ingredients 32

Preparation 32

Baked Apples 33

Ingredients 33

Preparation 33

Apple Cinnamon Breakfast Risotto 34

Ingredients 34

Preparation 34

Pumpkins Cinnamon Buns 35

Ingredients 35

Preparation 36

French Toast Casserole 37

Ingredients 37

Preparation 37

Hot Chocolate Oatmeal 39

Ingredients 39

Preparation 39

Spinach and Mozzarella Frittata 40

Ingredients 40

Preparation 40

Breakfast Casserole 41

Ingredients 41

Preparation 41

Blueberry-Chia Quinoa 42

Ingredients 42

Preparation 42

Almond-Cherry-Coconut Granola 43

Ingredients 43

Preparation 43

Two-Bean Beef Chili 44

Ingredients 44

Preparation 44

Root Vegetable Stew 45

Ingredients 45

Preparation 46

Lumberjack Vegetable Soup 47

Ingredients 47

Preparation 47

Chicken Tortilla Soup 48

Ingredients 48

Preparation 48

Chicken Pho 49

Ingredients 49

Preparation 49

Spicy Black Bean Soup 51

Ingredients 51

Preparation 51

Lentil and Sweet Potato Soup 53

Ingredients 53

Preparation 53

Cajun Stew 54

Ingredients 54

Preparation 54

Squash, Chickpea, and Red Lentil Stew 55

Ingredients 55

Preparation 55

Curried Carrot Soup 57

Ingredients 57

Preparation 57

Chinese Pork and Vegetable Hot Pot 59

Ingredients 59

Preparation 60

Mini Turkey Meatballs 61

Ingredients 61

Preparation 61

Pork Tacos 63

Ingredients 63

Preparation 63

Meaty Red Beans and Rice 65

Ingredients 65

Preparation 66

Chicken Stroganoff 67

Ingredients 67

Preparation 67

BBQ Beef Sandwiches 68

Ingredients 68

Preparation 68

Buffalo Chicken Lettuce Wraps 69

Ingredients 69

Preparation 69

Honey Sesame Chicken 70

Ingredients 70

Preparation 70

Rancher's Roast Beef 72

Ingredients 72

Preparation 72

Coconut Curry Chicken 73

Ingredients 73

Preparation 73

Pulled Pork 75

Ingredients 75

Preparation 75

Wine and Tomato Braised Chicken 77

Ingredients 77

Preparation 77

Hungarian Beef Goulash 79

Ingredients 79

Preparation 79

Stuffed Peppers 81

Ingredients 81

Preparation 81

Turkey Osso Buco 82

Ingredients 82

Preparation 82

Moroccan Lamb 83

Ingredients 83

Preparation 83

Shrimp and Artichoke Barley Risotto 85

Ingredients 85

Preparation 85

Cedar Plank Salmon 87

Ingredients 87

Preparation 87

Loaded Baked Potatos 88

Ingredients 88

Preparation 88

Vegetarian Tamale Pie 89

Ingredients 89

Preparation 89

Barley Risotto with Fennel 90

Ingredients 90

Preparation 90

Vegetarian Lasagna 92

Ingredients 92

Preparation 92

Vegetable Curry 94

Ingredients 94

Preparation 94

Garlic Cauliflower Mashed "Potatoes" 95

Ingredients 95

Preparation 95

Ratatouille 96

Ingredients 96

Preparation 96

Squash Lasagna 98

Ingredients 98

Preparation 98

Indian Chole 99

Ingredients 99

Preparation 99

Banana Brown Betty 100

Ingredients 100

Preparation 100

Poached Pears with Caramel Sauce 101

Ingredients 101

Preparation 101

Clean Eating Brownies 102

Ingredients 102

Preparation 102

Pumpkin Bread 104

Ingredients 104

Preparation 104

Chocolate Fudge 106

Ingredients 106

Preparation 106

Brown Rice Pudding 107

Ingredients 107

Preparation 107

Cranberry Sauce

Prep time: 10 mins

Total time: 2 hours 10 mins

Ingredients

- 12 ounces fresh cranberries
- 2 medium oranges (about ½ pound each)
- 1 medium apple (1/2 pound)
- ¾ cup maple syrup

Preparation

1. Rinse the cranberries and place them in the slow cooker.
2. Squeeze the juice out of one orange and add the juice to the slow cooker. (This is about ¼ cup of juice.)
3. Remove the peel from the second orange and chop the fruit into bite-sized pieces. Add them to the slow cooker.
4. Peel the apple and remove the core. Chop the apple into bite-sized pieces and add them to the slow cooker.
5. Add the maple syrup to the fruit and stir.
6. Turn on the slow cooker to "Low" and cook until the fruit is very tender. For me, this takes about 2 hours, but your slow cooker might take more or less time. Keep an eye on it.
7. Mash the fruit so there are no large chunks remaining. I use a potato masher, but you could also use a large spoon or fork (just don't scratch the slow cooker).
8. Turn the heat to high, and cook uncovered for an additional 15 minutes to thicken the sauce.
9. Serve the slow cooker cranberry sauce warm, or let the sauce cool and store it in an airtight container in the refrigerator until ready to serve.

Fig Apple Butter

Prep Time: 20 mins

Cook time: 8 hours

Total time: 8 hours 20 mins

Ingredients

- 20 dried black figs, stems removed, cut in half
- 6 apples, peeled, cored and diced
- 1 cup apple cider
- ½ cup honey (or other sweetener such as maple syrup)
- 3 tablespoons cinnamon (sounds like a lot, because it is, and it's awesome)
- ½ teaspoon ground cloves
- ¼ teaspoon nutmeg
- pinch of salt

Preparation

1. Place all ingredients in the slow cooker. Mix well.
2. Put the slow cooker at low and cook for 6-8 hours until apples are completely soft and almost mushy.
3. Place ingredients (I did mine in two batches) in food processor and puree until smooth.
4. Eat with anything. A spoon, on some banana bread, on a banana. Possibilities are endless.
5. Store in refrigerator in a jar. Because jars are cute.

Fruit and Berry Cobbler

Ingredients

Cobbler:

- 8 ounces frozen mango slices
- 8 ounces frozen mixed berries
- 1/2 cup pomegranate juice
- 1/2 tablespoon cornstarch
- 1/2 teaspoon pure vanilla extract

Topping:

- 1/2 cup rolled oats
- 1/4 cup flour
- 1/4-1/2 cup brown sugar
- 1 teaspoon baking powder
- salt
- 4 tablespoons unsalted butter, cold, cut into pieces

Preparation

1. Spray a 3 ½ quart slow cooker with cooking spray.
2. Place the frozen fruit in the bottom of the slow cooker.
3. Mix together the pomegranate juice, cornstarch, and vanilla; pour over the frozen fruit.
4. In a medium bowl, mix together the oats, flour, brown sugar, baking powder, and salt. Use your fingers to mix the butter into the dry ingredients, until the butter is broken into small pieces. Sprinkle the mixture over the fruit.
5. Place 3-4 layers of paper towels over the top of the slow cooker and place the lid on top (this will catch any steam

created by the slow cooker during cooking and prevent your topping from getting soggy).
6. Cook on low for 4-5 hours, or until the juices are thick and bubbly. Make sure not to lift the lid on the slow cooker for the first 3 hours of cooking.
7. Serve warm with your favorite vanilla ice cream.

Greek Yogurt

Ingredients

- 8 cups (half-gallon) of whole, 1%, 2% or skim Pasteurized Milk. Do NOT use ultra-pasteurized

- 1/2 cup store-bought natural plain yogurt. (Once you have made your own, you can use that as a starter)

Preparation

1. Add a half gallon of milk to crock pot. Cover and cook on LOW for approximately 2 1/2 hours. Using a candy thermometer, check the temperature of the milk. When the milk has reached 180 degrees, unplug the crock pot, remove the cover, and let it sit for another hour or so. You are waiting for the milk to come down in temperature to between 105 and 110 degrees.
2. When the milk has reached that temp, scoop out 1 to 2 cups of the warmish milk and whisk in 1/2 cup of store-bought yogurt. Then pour the mixture back into the crock pot. Wisk to combine.
3. At this point I added 3/4 cup honey. I am not a fan of PLAIN yogurt, Greek or otherwise, and since my favorite store-bought variety is honey flavored, I thought I would make my homemade kind honey flavored as well.
4. Put the lid back on your crock pot, wrap a heavy bath towel around the crock for insulation, and place in the oven with the oven light ON.
5. Leave the yogurt undisturbed for 7 or 8 hours, or overnight.
6. In the morning, carefully take the crock out, unwrap it and remove the lid, and check to see whether the milk has turned to yogurt.
7. (If your batch isn't quite thickened, return it to the oven and check on it again in an hour.)

8. Now here's the part that makes it GREEK yogurt: refrigerate the yogurt for at least three hours to allow it to completely cool and thicken. Line a large strainer with four layers of damp cheesecloth and put inside a bowl. Pour the yogurt in; refrigerate for one hour. Pour out the liquid that has accumulated in the bottom of the bowl; this is the whey. Return the bowl to the refrigerator for one more hour, strain the liquid again and the yogurt should now look thick and creamy.

Paleo Slow Cooker Ketchup

Prep time: 15 mins

Cook time: 10 hours

Total time: 10 hours 15 mins

Ingredients

- 5 lbs of Ripe Tomatoes (stewing tomatoes) or 2 (28 oz) cans of Crushed Tomatoes
- 1 cup of Dried Medjool Dates (about 22), pitted and peeled
- ¾ cup of White Vinegar
- 2 Tablespoons of Kosher Salt
- ½ teaspoon of All Spice
- ½ teaspoon of Black Pepper
- ½ teaspoon of Garlic Powder
- ½ teaspoon of Onion Powder
- ½ teaspoon of Mustard Powder
- ¼ teaspoon of Ginger Powder
- ¼ teaspoon of Mace
- 3 Whole Cloves or ¼ teaspoon of Ground Cloves

Preparation

1. Cut off the stem pits from the tomatoes. If using canned tomatoes, just add them directly to the crock pot and proceed to step five.
2. Blanch the tomatoes by dropping them in boiling water for a minute. Peel them when they are cool enough to touch.

3. Slice the peeled tomatoes in half and remove the liquid and seeds. No need to squeeze them.
4. Transfer the cored tomatoes to the crock pot.
5. Add the dates, vinegar, salt, and spices except the cloves to the pot.
6. Blend together with an immersion blend and add the cloves.
7. Cook on high uncovered for about 8-10 hours until sauce has reduced by half and is thick and pasty. This needs to be monitored and stirred every few hours.
8. Blend the sauce with an immersion blender once again
9. Strain the sauce with a mesh sieve to remove the chunky bits.
10. Adjust seasoning and enjoy!

Pumpkin Butter

Prep Time: 5 minutes

Cook Time: 5 hours

Total Time: 5 hours, 5 minutes

Yield: approximately 10 ounces

Ingredients

- 4 cups of pumpkin (approximately 2 15 ounce cans, or use your own pumpkin purée)
- 1 1/4 cup maple syrup or honey (sugar works, too, but we are reducing our sugar intake)
- 2 t cinnamon
- 1 t ground ginger
- 1/2 t nutmeg
- 1 t vanilla extract, optional

Preparation

1. Mix together pumpkin purée, maple syrup (or other sweetener), and vanilla (if you are using it) in the crock-pot.
2. Cover, and cook on high for 4 hours or overnight on low for 8 hours.
3. In the last hour of cooking, add the cinnamon, ginger, and nutmeg, and crack the lid to let moisture out if you want a thicker consistency.
4. Cool and store in jars at the bottom of your fridge.

Paleo Pumpkin Pie Pudding

Ingredients

- 3 tbs. melted coconut oil or butter
- 3 cups pureed pumpkin
- 2 cups coconut milk
- 3 eggs
- 1/3-1/2 cup natural sweetener of choice (I used a mixture of palm sugar and maple syrup)
- 2 tsp. pumpkin pie spice
- 1.5 tbs. vanilla extract
- 3 tbs. coconut flour
- 1 tsp. baking powder

Preparation

1. Use a little of the melted coconut oil or butter to grease the inside of the crock pot. Then add all ingredients and stir to combine. If you want a really even, creamy texture you can whip it all up in a blender or use a stick blender right in the crock pot first. I just used a lot of elbow grease until the pumpkin lumps were smoothed out.
2. Cover crock pot and cook on low for 6-8 hours. Pudding will get a crust on top and start to brown on edges (as shown below), but still be pudding-like underneath.

Spiced Hot Apple Cidar

Ingredients

- 2 Cinnamon Sticks
- 1 tablespoon Clove
- 1/2 teaspoon Allspice
- 2 quarts organic 100% apple juice (fresh juiced if possible)
- 1 lemon, thinly sliced
- 1 orange, thinly sliced

Preparation

1. Juice apples for 2 qts of juice
2. Combine 1 cup apple juice and spices in large dutch oven, boil then simmer 10 minutes
3. Strain the cinnamon sticks out and then return the liquid to dutch oven. Combine with lemon & orange
4. Cook over low heat until thoroughly heated.
5. Serve warm

Strawberry Applesauce

Ingredients

- about 6-7 cups peeled, cored and sliced apples- any variety
- 1 pound container strawberries, stems removed
- 1/2 cup water
- sugar to taste (raw, white, or brown) I used 3 tablespoons of sugar in the raw

Preparation

1. Add the apples and strawberries to a 5-quart or larger slow cooker. Add the water.
2. Cover, and cook on HIGH for 4 hours.
3. Add cooked apples and strawberries to a blender, cover and pulse just a few times until smooth but not pulverized.
4. Stir in the sugar to taste.
5. Serve and enjoy!

Vanilla Bean Honeycrisp Applesauce

Prep time: 20 mins

Cook time: 4 hours

Total time: 4 hours 20 mins

Ingredients

- 5 large honeycrisp apples, peeled, cored and thinly sliced
- 1 lemon
- 1 cinnamon stick
- 1 vanilla bean

Preparation

1. Put apple slices in large slow cooker.
2. Juice lemon, pour over apples, and toss to coat.
3. Add cinnamon stick to slow cooker.
4. Split vanilla bean and scrap seeds with knife. Add bean pod and scraped seeds to slow cooker.
5. Cover and cook on high for 4 hours. There should be no need to add water. When done, stir with large spoon to achieve desired consistency.
6. Can in water bath for storage or store in refrigerator in airtight container up to 2 weeks.

Yogurt, Kid-Made!

Prep time: 30 mins

Cook time: 4 hours

Total time: 4 hours 30 mins

Serves: 6

Ingredients

- ½ Gallon Whole Organic Milk
- ½ Cup Plain Yogurt

Preparation

1. A half gallon of milk goes into your slow cooker.
2. Insert a cooking thermometer into the cooker and tie it up, so it doesn't slip inside.
3. Click "boil" on the slow cooker and stir the milk to prevent it from scalding as the liquid heats.
4. Watch the temperature. When it reaches 200 degrees, turn the slow cooker off.
5. Then scoop an unmeasured cup of the milk from the slow cooker and pour it into a medium sized mixing bowl. As a half cup of pre-made plain yogurt and stir the two together.
6. Wait until the milk returns to 112 degrees. Then pour the milk/yogurt mixture back into the slow cooker and whisk it all until well combined.
7. Cover the slow cooker, pile on some blankets and wait.
8. Four hours later, your yogurt is ready to transfer to the refrigerator. You can pour it into a jar and place in the cold. As it chills, it will set.

Cinnamon Apple Oatmeal

Ingredients

- Non-stick cooking spray
- 2 large tart apples (such as Granny Smith or Pink Lady), chopped
- 1 1/2 cups skim milk
- 1 1/2 cups water
- 1 cup whole grain oats
- 3 tablespoons packed dark brown sugar
- 2 tablespoons butter
- 1 tablespoon cinnamon (more or less to your taste)
- 2 tablespoons milled/ground flaxseed
- 1/4 teaspoon kosher salt
- Additional Topping:
- 1/4 cup dried fruit (raisins, cranberries)
- 1/4 cup chopped nuts (walnuts, almonds, pecans)

Preparation

1. Spray a 3 1/2 quart or larger slow cooker with non-stick cooking spray. Combine chopped apples, milk, water, oats, sugar, butter, and flax- stirring to combine. Cover and cook on low for 7-8 hours (overnight). Stir in 1/4 teaspoon kosher salt into the oatmeal just before serving.
2. If desired, serve with additional toppings (1 tablespoon dried fruit and 1 tablespoon chopped nuts, each)

Banana Bread Quinoa

Ingredients

- 1 cup of quinoa (I used Bob's Red Mill)
- 1/2 cup of Seasonal Coffee-mate Warm Cinnamon Sugar Cookie •
- 1/2 cup low-fat milk
- 1 cup water
- 1 1/2 banana (past ripe)
- 2 tablespoons chopped walnuts
- 3 tablespoons brown sugar
- 1 1/2 tablespoons butter, melted
- 1/2 teaspoon vanilla extract

Preparation

1. Mash the banana in a bowl and set aside. In another bowl, mix the brown sugar and walnuts together.
2. Pour quinoa, creamer (or light cream), milk, water, butter and vanilla into the crock pot. Add the mashed banana and stir to evenly distribute. Sprinkle the sugar and walnut mixture into the quinoa and stir to mix.
3. Cook on low for 4 – 6 hours, or until the quinoa is fully cooked. If you need to, add additional liquid or sugar to the mixture for taste.
4. Serve warm and garish with slices of banana!

Vegetable Breakfast Burritos

Ingredients

- 1 15oz can black beans, drained and rinsed
- 1 10oz can diced tomatoes with green chiles, don't drain
- 1 cup uncooked pearl barley
- 2 cups vegetable broth
- 3/4 cups frozen corn, no need to thaw
- 1/4 cup chopped green onions
- 1 tablespoon fresh squeezed lime juice
- 1 teaspoon ground cumin
- 1 teaspoon chili powder
- 1/2 teaspoon ground red pepper
- 3 garlic cloves, chopped

Preparation

1. Place the following in a crockpot, give it all a stir, and set the pot on low. Cook for 4-5 hours (I usually go for 5).
2. When the filling is done, scramble however many eggs you intend to eat, and spread some of the filling on an flour tortilla along with the eggs. Garnish with any or all of the following:
3. Shredded cheddar cheese
4. Fresh cilantro
5. Salsa
6. Lettuce
7. Guacamole

Greek Yogurt

Ingredients

- 1/2 gallon milk (you can really use however much you like.)
- 1/2 cup of plain yogurt (for a starter, to get the process going)
- 1/4 cup powdered milk. (optional)
- crock pot
- thermometer
- blanket
- colander and cheesecloth if you are going to make greek yogurt

Preparation

1. Pour your milk in your crock pot and set it on high.
2. Heat milk until it reaches 180° (this took about 2 hours for me. If you have a nicer crock pot it might be quicker)
3. When 180° is reached, unplug crock pot, take the lid off and let cool until it's around 110°.
4. In a separate small bowl, mix together plain yogurt and powdered milk (if using)
5. When the temp is around 110°, add yogurt mixture and stir well.
6. Place the lid back on, and wrap crock pot in a blanket like a little yogurt baby, and let it sit on the counter for about 6 hours.
7. You now have yogurt!
8. You'll notice a watery substance on top, this is they whey.
9. You can mix it in, and put your yogurt in the fridge and it's ready to eat as soon as it's chilled.

Baked Apples

Ingredients

- 6 medium to large green apples
- ¼ cup raisins
- ¼ cup honey
- 1 teaspoon cinnamon
- 6 tablespoons coconut oil, butter, or ghee

Preparation

1. Core apples. To core, using an apple corer or paring knife, cut around the core (about ¼ inch from the stem all the way around) but leave about half an inch at the bottom. Use the knife to 'drill out' the core.
2. Divide raisins, honey, cinnamon, and coconut oil between the apples.
3. Place apples in a crock pot and add ½ inch of water. Cook on low overnight and enjoy a hot breakfast in the morning!
4. Alternatively, bake covered at 350 degrees in a glass dish for 45 minutes-1 hour in the morning.
5. Top with with cream, yogurt, coconut milk, or just eat plain.

Apple Cinnamon Breakfast Risotto

Ingredients

- 1/4 cup butter
- 3 little apples (I had 2 greens, and 1 red in the house)
- 1 1/2 t cinnamon
- 1/8 t nutmeg
- 1/8 t cloves
- 1/4 t kosher salt
- 1 1/2 cups arborio rice
- 1/3 cup brown sugar
- 4 cups of liquid.

Preparation

1. I used a 4 qt round crockpot for this dish.
2. Turn your crock to high and add the butter so it can start melting. Wash and cut up your apples while it begins to melt.
3. Add the rice to the butter, and stir it around to coat it nicely. If the butter isn't completely melted, don't worry. Mine wasn't either, and it didn't seem to make a difference.
4. Add the apples, and spices. Stir in the juice/milk.
5. Cover and cook on high for 3-5 hours, or on low for 6 or so.
6. I was really surprised how long it took---I needed to cook it on high for 4.5 hours---and since I just made the rice and beans, I thought it would cook as fast as that dish did.

Pumpkins Cinnamon Buns

Ingredients

- 3 cups all purpose flour
- 1/4 cup sugar
- 1 package active dry yeast
- 1/2 cup vanilla almond milk
- 1/4 cup water
- 3/4 cup pureed pumpkin
- 1/2 cup canola oil
- 1 Flaxseed egg (1 TBS flaxseed to 1 1/2 TBS warm water, let it sit for 5 minutes)

Filling Ingredients:

- 1/3 cup butter
- 1/3 cup brown sugar
- 2 tsp ground cinnamon
- 2 tsp nutmeg
- 1 tsp ginger
- 1 tsp ground gloves
- Icing Ingredients:
- 4 oz vegan cream cheese, soft
- 1 cup powdered sugar
- 1/2 stick vegan butter, soft
- 1/2 tsp vanilla extract
- 1/2 tsp lemon juice

Preparation

1. In a large bowl, combine flour, sugar and yeast. Fold in almond milk, water, pumpkin, flaxseed egg and oil into try ingredients. Form into a ball and let it sit in bowl, covered with a towel, for 30-45 minutes.
2. Once dough has settled, roll into a rectangle on a lightly floured surface.
3. Mix together filling ingredients and baste rolled rectangle dough with sugary, pumpkin spice mixture. Roll long side to long side, pinch ends and then cut into 12-14 slices.
4. Place in greased crock pot and cook on high for 60-90 minutes (perform the toothpick test to determine doneness. If it comes out clean, you're good to go!)
5. Mix up icing/glaze and pour over hot rolls to create an ooey, gooey, perfectly moist cinnamon bun. Top with pecan pieces if you're feeling wild.

French Toast Casserole
Ingredients

- 2 whole eggs
- 2 egg whites
- 1 1/2 cups 1% milk, (almond or soy will also work)
- 2 tablespoon honey
- 1 teaspoon vanilla extract
- 1/2 teaspoon cinnamon
- 9 Slices whole grain bread

FILLING:

- 3 cups finely diced uncooked apple pieces (Honey Crisp or Gala are both great in this recipe)
- 3 tablespoon honey
- 1 teaspoon lemon juice
- 1/3 cup diced raw pecans
- 1/2 teaspoon cinnamon

Preparation

1. Add the first 6 ingredients to a medium mixing bowl, whisk to combine. Lightly spray the inside of the slow cooker with nonstick cooking spray.
2. Add all the filling ingredients in a small mixing bowl and stir to coat apple pieces, set aside.
3. Cut bread slices into triangles (that's in half, just triangle shaped). Place one layer of bread (6 triangles) on the bottom of the slow cooker, add ¼ of the filling and repeat until there are 3 layers of bread. Add the remaining filling to the top.

4. Pour egg mixture over bread. Cover and cook on high 2 to 2-1/2 or low 4 hours, or until bread has soaked up the liquid.
5. 3 Bananas (diced) can be substituted for apples.
6. Note: Drizzle with 100% pure maple syrup if desired.

Hot Chocolate Oatmeal

Ingredients

- 1 c. steel-cut oats
- 4 c. water
- 1/2 c. coconut milk

- 1 T. cocoa powder
- 1 t. vanilla
- 1/4 t. salt
- 1 T. coconut palm sugar or pure maple syrup
- 8 drops liquid stevia (or an extra tablespoon of sugar)

Preparation

1. In a large bowl, combine the water, milk, vanilla, and stevia. Whisk in the cocoa, sugar, and salt.
2. Finally, stir in the oats. Oil the inside of your slow cooker (this prevents the oatmeal from sticking). Pour in the above mixture.
3. Set your slow cooker to LOW for 1-2 hours, and turn it to KEEP WARM before finally retiring to bed. In the morning, give it all a stir and feast! Top with some shaved chocolate if you're feeling really decadent!
4. Makes 4 Servings

Spinach and Mozzarella Frittata

Ingredients

- 1 tablespoon extra virgin olive oil
- 1/2 cup diced onion
- 1 cup 2% shredded mozzarella cheese, divided
- 3 eggs
- 3 egg whites
- 2 tablespoons 1% milk
- 1/4 teaspoon black pepper
- 1/4 teaspoon white pepper
- 1 (packed) cup chopped baby spinach, with stems removed
- 1 Roma tomato, diced
- Salt to taste

Preparation

1. In a small skillet, add oil and sauté onion on medium heat until tender, about 5 minutes.
2. Lightly spray the inside of the slow cooker with nonstick cooking spray. We like to make our own by filling this reusable cooking spray bottle with olive oil or canola oil.
3. In a large bowl, combine sautéed onion, 3/4 cup mozzarella cheese, and remaining ingredients; whisk to combine, and pour into slow cooker. Sprinkle remaining 1/4 cup cheese on top of egg mixture. Cover, and cook on LOW for 1–1 1/2 hours, or until eggs are set and a knife inserted in the center comes out clean.

Breakfast Casserole
Ingredients

- 1 dozen eggs
- 1 cup cup nonfat milk
- 1 package (32 oz) hash browns
- 1 lb turkey bacon, cut into pieces
- 1/2 cup green onions
- 1 green, red, or yellow pepper, diced
- 1/2 lb reduced-fat jalapeno jack cheese, shredded or cut in pieces
- salt and pepper to taste

Preparation

1. Layer potatoes, bacon, onions, pepper and cheese in the crock pot in two or three layers
2. Beat the eggs, milk, and salt and pepper together.
3. Pour over entire mixture.
4. Cook with crock pot on low for 10 hours until eggs set and are thoroughly cooked.

Blueberry-Chia Quinoa

Prep time: 5 mins

Cook time: 6 hours

Total time: 6 hours 5 mins

Ingredients

- 4 cups soy milk
- 4 cups water
- 2 cups quinoa
- 2 cups blueberries
- 1/3 cup chia seeds
- 1/3 cup honey

Preparation

1. Stir soy milk, water, quinoa, blueberries, chia seeds, and honey together in a slow cooker.
2. Cook on Low 6 to 8 hours.

Almond-Cherry-Coconut Granola

Ingredients

- 5 cups old fashioned rolled oats
- 1 cup raw, whole almonds
- 1/2 cup dried tart cherries
- 1/2 cup pepitas (unsalted hulled pumpkin seeds)
- 1/4 cup unsweetened shredded coconut
- 1/4 cup canola oil
- 1/4 cup honey
- 1 teaspoon vanilla

Preparation

Slow cooker instructions:

1. Place the oats, honey, oil, vanilla, almonds and vanilla in a 4 quart slow cooker. Stir. Leave uncovered and turn on high. Cook for 1 hour, stirring every 20 to 30minutes. Reduce to low and add the coconut, pepitas and cherries. Continued to cook on low uncovered for about 4 hours, stirring every 20 or so minutes. The granola is done when it looks completely dry. Cool on baking sheets then store in an air tight container.

Oven instructions:

1. Preheat oven to 250. In a large bowl, combine all ingredients but the dried cherries. Divide among 3 baking sheets and spread to a thin layer. Cook for 1 hour and 15 minutes, stirring every 15 minutes. Pour it back into the bowl, and stir in the cherries. Allow to cool on baking sheets then store in an air tight container.

Two-Bean Beef Chili

Ingredients

- 1 lb ground beef
- 2 cans precooked beans of choice, drained
- 3 to 4 cans diced canned tomatoes with liquid (or plain tomato sauce, or mixture of both)
- 1 large white onion, diced
- 1 TBSP olive oil
- Salt + pepper to taste
- Cumin to taste, approx. 2 teaspoons or to taste
- Chili powder to taste (approx. 1/4 cup)
- 1 teaspoon sugar, optional
- Garlic powder to taste
- Garlic salt, optional
- Cayenne pepper, approx. 1/2 teaspoon or to taste

Preparation

1. In nonstick skillet, cook onions in olive oil until softened; add to crock pot. •Important to cook down onions before adding in tomatoes which could hamper cooking.
2. Add in all other ingredients, break beef up with spoon; cook on medium-high for 4-6 hours or until beef is cooked thoroughly. Stir every so often.

Root Vegetable Stew

Total Time: 30 mins, plus 3 1/2 hrs cooking time

Active Time: 30 mins

Makes: 6 to 8 servings

Ingredients

- 1/4 cup olive oil
- 2 medium yellow onions, large dice
- Kosher salt
- 1 1/4 teaspoons ground ginger
- 1 (3-inch) cinnamon stick
- 1/2 teaspoon ground coriander
- 1/4 teaspoon ground cumin
- 1/8 teaspoon cayenne pepper
- Pinch saffron threads
- Freshly ground black pepper
- 1 pound Yukon Gold potatoes (about 3 large), large dice
- 1 pound carrots (about 4 to 5 medium), peeled and large dice
- 1 pound parsnips (about 4 medium), peeled and large dice
- 3 cups low-sodium chicken or vegetable broth
- 2 pounds sugar baby pumpkin or butternut squash (about 1 small), peeled, seeded, and large dice
- 1 pound sweet potatoes (about 2 medium), peeled and large dice
- 1 (15-ounce) can chickpeas, also known as garbanzo beans, drained and rinsed (about 1 1/2 cups)

- 1/2 cup golden raisins, also known as sultanas
- 1 bunch spinach, trimmed and washed (about 4 cups loosely packed)
- 1 1/2 tablespoons cider vinegar, plus more as needed

Preparation

1. Heat the oil in a large frying pan over medium heat until shimmering. Add the onions and a pinch of salt and cook over medium heat until translucent, about 4 minutes. Add the ginger, cinnamon, coriander, cumin, cayenne, saffron, and a pinch of pepper and cook until fragrant, about 1 minute.
2. Transfer the mixture to a slow cooker, add the potatoes, carrots, parsnips, and broth, season with salt and pepper, and stir to combine. Cover and cook on high for 1 1/2 hours.
3. Add the pumpkin or squash, sweet potatoes, chickpeas, and raisins, season with salt, and stir to combine. Cover and continue to cook on high until a knife easily pierces the vegetables, about 2 hours more, stirring after 1 hour. Add the spinach and gently mix (do not overmix). Let sit until wilted. Gently stir in the vinegar, taste, and season with more salt, pepper, and vinegar as needed.

Lumberjack Vegetable Soup

Ingredients

- 7 ½ cups chopped rutabaga
- 6 cups chopped carrots
- 1 ½ cups chopped celery
- 1 ½ cups chopped mushrooms
- 18 cups water
- 2 cups cooked chickpeas (roast for 15 to 20 minutes at 350 degrees)
- 5 teaspoons garlic powder
- 2 tablespoon black pepper
- 1 cup organic Dijon mustard
- 1 tablespoons extra-virgin olive oil
- 1 tablespoon sea salt
- 2 low sodium vegetable bullion cubes
- 6 cups fresh spinach

Preparation

1. Place all ingredients except spinach in a slow cooker. Cook for approximately 6 hours until rutabaga and carrots are soft. Add spinach, allow to cook down, stir to incorporate into soup.

Chicken Tortilla Soup

Ingredients

- 4 chicken breast halves
- 2 (15 ounce) cans black beans, undrained
- 2 (15 ounce) cans stewed tomatoes
- 1 cup salsa
- 15 ounces tomato sauce
- tortilla chips
- 1 cup shredded cheese

Preparation

1. Combine everything except chips and cheese in crockpot. Cook on low for 8 hours.
2. Before serving, remove chicken and cut into bite size pieces. Put chips in bowls, top with soup and sprinkle with cheese. (But it is also good straight.).
3. Make a double batch. You'll want it.

Chicken Pho

Ingredients

- 2 pounds chicken parts (recommend of the 2 pounds, use 1/2 pound chicken wing tips)
- 1/2 onion
- 3-inch chunk of ginger, sliced
- 2 tablespoons whole coriander seeds
- 4 whole cloves
- 2 whole star anise
- 2 tablespoons sugar (or rock sugar)
- 2 tablespoons fish sauce
- Small bunch of cilantro stems, tied in bunch with twine
- 1 pound dried rice noodles (about 1/4" wide)
- 1/2 pound chicken meat (breast or thigh), thinly sliced
- 2 cups bean sprouts, washed
- Handful of cilantro leaves
- 1/2 cup shaved red onions
- 1/2 lime, cut into 4 wedges
- Sriracha hot sauce (optional)
- Hoisin sauce (optional)

Preparation

1. To the slow cooker, add the chicken, onion, ginger, coriander seeds, cloves, star anise, sugar, fish sauce, and cilantro stems. Fill with water to the max level of your slow cooker. Turn slow cooker to high for 4-6 hours or low for 8-10

hours. Remove all chicken and cilantro stems, strain broth through cheesecloth. Taste and adjust with additional fish sauce and sugar if needed.
2. Soak rice noodles in cool water for 5 minutes. Drain. In the meantime, bring a big pot of water to a boil and then turn to low. Add the chicken slices and let cook for 1-3 minutes or until cooked through–timing depends on how thin slices are. Remove the chicken slices. Next, add the rice noodles to the water and cook for 1 minute. Remove noodles and divide amongst 4 serving bowls.
3. Fill each bowl with chicken slices, bean sprouts, cilantro leaves, red onions and broth. Have the lime, Sriracha and hoisin at table as condiments.

Spicy Black Bean Soup

Ingredients

- 1 tablespoon olive oil
- 2 medium-size red onions, chopped
- 1 medium-size red bell pepper, chopped
- 1 medium-size green bell pepper, chopped
- 4 garlic cloves, minced
- 4 teaspoons ground cumin
- 1 16-ounce package dried black beans
- 1 tablespoon chopped chipotle chiles from a can (use less if you prefer less heat)
- 7 cups hot water (tap water is fine)
- 2 tablespoons fresh lime juice
- 2 teaspoons coarse kosher salt
- 1/4 teaspoon ground black pepper
- Optional toppings:
- sour cream
- greek yogurt
- crema or creme fraiche
- avocado

Preparation

1. Heat olive oil in large skillet over medium-high heat. Add onions and both bell peppers and sauté until beginning to brown, about eight minutes. Add garlic and cumin; stir one minute. Transfer mixture to 6-quart slow cooker. Add beans

and chipotles, then 7 cups hot water. Cover and cook on high until beans are very tender, about 3 hours, but longer if necessary. [See note up top.]
2. Transfer four cups bean mixture to blender; puree until smooth. Return puree to remaining soup in slow cooker. Stir in lime juice, salt, and pepper. Adjust seasonings to taste. Ladle soup into bowls. Serve with desired toppings.
3. Per serving: calories, 314; total fat, 4 g; saturated fat, 1 g; cholesterol, 1 mg; fiber, 18 g

Lentil and Sweet Potato Soup

Time: 10 hours

Ingredients

- 4 large carrots, chopped
- 4 stalks celery, chopped
- 1 onion, diced
- 2 large sweet potatoes, peeled and cubed
- 1.5 cups chopped green beans
- 2 cups green lentils
- 1 tsp minced fresh rosemary
- 1 bay leaf
- 1 tsp dried oregano
- 4 cloves garlic, minced
- 1 15-oz can diced tomatoes
- 64 oz vegetable broth
- 2 tsp salt (or to taste)
- 1/2 tsp pepper

Preparation

1. Combine all ingredients in a slow cooker. Turn heat on low and cook for 10 hours, adding a little more broth at the end if soup seems too thick.

Cajun Stew

Ingredients

- 3/4 pound andouille or kielbasa, sliced into 1/2-inch-thick rounds
- 1 red onion, sliced into wedges
- 2 garlic cloves, minced
- 2 celery stalks, coarsely chopped
- 1 red or green bell pepper, coarsely chopped
- 2 tablespoons all-purpose flour
- 1 (28-ounce) can diced tomatoes
- 1/4 teaspoon cayenne pepper
- Coarse salt
- 1/2 pound large shrimp, peeled and deveined
- 2 cups frozen cut okra (from an 8-ounce package), thawed

Preparation

1. In a 5-to-6-quart slow cooker, place sausage, onion, garlic, celery, and bell pepper. Sprinkle with flour and toss to coat. Add tomatoes and their liquid, 1/2 cup water, and cayenne; season with salt. Cover and cook until vegetables are tender, 3 1/2 hours on high (or 7 hours on low). Add shrimp and okra, cover, and cook until shrimp are opaque throughout, 30 minutes (or 1 hour on low).

Squash, Chickpea, and Red Lentil Stew

Ingredients

- 3/4 cup dried chickpeas
- 2 1/2 pounds kabocha squash, (see Note) or butternut squash, peeled, seeded and cut into 1-inch cubes
- 2 large carrots, peeled and cut into 1/2-inch pieces
- 1 large onion, chopped
- 1 cup red lentils
- 4 cups vegetable broth
- 2 tablespoons tomato paste
- 1 tablespoon minced peeled fresh ginger
- 1 1/2 teaspoons ground cumin
- 1 teaspoon salt
- 1/4 teaspoon saffron, (see Note)
- 1/4 teaspoon freshly ground pepper
- 1/4 cup lime juice
- 1/2 cup chopped roasted unsalted peanuts
- 1/4 cup packed fresh cilantro leaves, chopped

Preparation

1. Soak chickpeas in enough cold water to cover them by 2 inches for 6 hours or overnight. (Alternatively, use the quick-soak method: Place beans in a large pot with enough water to cover by 2 inches. Bring to a boil over high heat. Remove from heat and let stand for 1 hour.) Drain when ready to use.

2. Combine the soaked chickpeas, squash, carrots, onion, lentils, broth, tomato paste, ginger, cumin, salt, saffron and pepper in a 6-quart slow cooker.
3. Put on the lid and cook on low until the chickpeas are tender and the lentils have begun to break down, 5 to 6 1/2 hours.
4. Stir in lime juice. Serve sprinkled with peanuts and cilantro.

Curried Carrot Soup

Ingredients

- Olive oil
- 1 clove garlic, chopped
- 1 to 2 teaspoons mild gluten-free curry powder, or to taste
- 1 leek
- 4 large organic carrots
- 1 sweet potato
- Half a banana squash {or butternut squash}
- Fresh water, as needed
- Sea salt, to taste

Preparation

1. Plug in your (medium size) slow cooker and turn it on to high. Pour a drizzle of olive oil into the bottom. Add in the chopped garlic and curry powder. Stir and cover. Let the curry infuse the oil as you chop the vegetables.
2. Wash the leek, trim and slice the white section.
3. Peel, trim and chop the carrots. Peel the sweet potato. Chop chop. Peel the squash. Chop some more.
4. Toss all the chopped veggies into the warm crock and stir. Add just enough fresh water to cover them. Season with sea salt to taste. Cover.
5. Now go to work. Or not. Maybe go do something fun. Take photographs. Paint. Read a gardening book. Walk the dog. Color with your kids.
6. About temps- High vs Low::
7. If you keep the soup on high it will cook faster- say, four hours or so, depending upon your make and model (some crocks are bigger than others, I'm happy to tell you). If you

need to stretch out the cooking time, turn the slow cooker on to low. It will be ready in perhaps, six hours. If you need to stretch it a bit longer I don't think it would hurt- as long as you've put enough water in the crock.

8. The soup is ready when the carrots are tender and split easily using a fork.
9. Now the fun part. Power tools.
10. Puree the soup with an immersion blender until the soup is silky smooth. Taste test. If it cooked down too much and is a tad thick, add some liquid {for extra creaminess use a dash of coconut milk- although- I didn't add any extra "milk" and we loved the fresh, clean taste} and gently heat through for another ten minutes.
11. Serve with pan toasted cornbread croutons.

Chinese Pork and Vegetable Hot Pot

Active Time: 40 minutes

Total Time: 3 3/4-6 3/4 hours

Ingredients

- 2 cups baby carrots
- 2 medium white turnips, (8 ounces total), peeled and cut into 3/4-inch-wide wedges
- 2 1/4 pounds boneless pork shoulder, (picnic or Boston-butt), trimmed and cut into 1 1/2-inch chunks
- 1 bunch scallions, sliced, white and green parts separated
- 1 14-ounce can reduced-sodium chicken broth
- 1/2 cup water
- 1/4 cup reduced-sodium soy sauce
- 3 tablespoons medium or dry sherry, (see Ingredient Note)
- 4 teaspoons brown sugar
- 2 tablespoons minced fresh ginger
- 1 tablespoon rice vinegar
- 2-4 teaspoons Chinese chile-garlic sauce
- 4 cloves garlic, minced
- 1 star anise pod, (see Ingredient Note) or 1 teaspoon aniseed
- 1 cinnamon stick
- 4 teaspoons cornstarch mixed with 2 tablespoons water
- 2 tablespoons toasted sesame seeds, (see Ingredient Note) for garnish

Preparation

1. Place carrots and turnips in the bottom and up the sides of a 4-quart or larger slow cooker. Top with pork and scallion whites. Bring broth, water, soy sauce, sherry, brown sugar, ginger, vinegar, chile-garlic sauce to taste and garlic to a simmer in a medium saucepan over medium-high heat. Pour over the pork and vegetables. Nestle star anise pod (or aniseed) and cinnamon stick into the stew. Cover and cook until the pork and vegetables are tender, 3 to 3 1/2 hours on high or 5 1/2 to 6 hours on low.
2. Discard the star anise pod and cinnamon stick. Skim or blot any visible fat from the surface of the stew. Add the cornstarch mixture, cover and cook on high, stirring 2 or 3 times, until slightly thickened, 10 to 15 minutes. Serve sprinkled with scallion greens and sesame seeds.

Mini Turkey Meatballs

Ingredients

- 1 pound 99% lean ground turkey breast
- 1 pound 94% lean ground turkey
- 2/3 cup cooked quinoa (preferably cooked in flavored stock)
- 3 garlic cloves, minced or pressed
- 1 large egg, lightly beaten
- 2 tablespoons olive oil
- 2 tablespoons finely grated romano cheese
- 2 teaspoons dried basil
- 1 teaspoon dried oregano
- 1/2 teaspoon onion powder
- 1/2 teaspoon salt
- 1/2 teaspoon pepper
- 1 large sweet onion, sliced into thin rounds
- 2 (28 ounce) cans crushed tomatoes

Preparation

1. In a large bowl, combine turkey, quinoa, garlic, beaten egg, olive oil, cheese, basil, oregano, salt and pepper. Mix thoroughly but quickly, just so the ingredients are combined - do not overmix! Roll into mini balls - slightly smaller than a golfball, and place on a baking sheet.
2. Layer sliced onion on the bottom of the crockpot and add 1 can of crushed tomatoes.
3. Heat a large skillet over medium-high heat (mine was actually almost high) and add 1/2 tablespoon olive oil. Add meatballs, searing on the top and bottom until golden, about

1 minute per side. To flip meatballs, gently toss with a spoon. I also shook the pan a few times to roll the meatballs around - if you pan is hot enough this works! Add meatballs one at a time to the crockpot. Repeat with remaining meatballs - it is okay to stack them once they are all finished.
4. Once all the meatballs are in the crockpot, add the other can of crushed tomatoes, completely submerging the meatballs. Cook on low for 6 hours. Serve!
5. {don't skip the browning step! it helps seal the juices in so the meatballs are tender and also keeps them from becoming one giant mess of meat in the crockpot.}
6. {if desired, you can brown the meatballs one day (such as the day before) and then refrigerate until ready to use. you can also freeze the same way!}

Pork Tacos

Ingredients

- 4-5lb pork butt (may be called pork shoulder)
- salt & pepper
- 1 large sweet onion
- 4 chipotle peppers in adobo sauce + 2 Tablespoons sauce
- 1/2 cup BBQ sauce
- 2 Tablespoons brown sugar
- 20oz Dr. Pepper
- Fajita-sized tortillas
- For the Cherry-Peach Salsa:
- 1 cup chopped sweet cherries
- 1 cup chopped peaches (about 1 large peach)
- 1/4 cup chopped cilantro
- 1 jalapeno, minced
- salt
- juice of 1 lime

Preparation

1. Cut onion into quarters then separate layers into the bottom of a 5 quart (minimum size) crock pot. Trim pork butt of excess fat then cut into 4-6 large pieces and season well with salt & pepper. Lay seasoned pork on top of onions then add chipotle peppers, adobo sauce, BBQ sauce, brown sugar, and Dr. Pepper. Cover and cook on low for 8 hours or until pork is tender enough to easily shred with a fork.

2. Remove pork pieces from the crock pot and shred, then place into a bowl and set aside. Strain juices through a double layer of cheesecloth and add back to shredded pork. Serve with Cherry-Peach Salsa in flour tortillas.
3. For the Cherry-Peach Salsa: Combine all ingredients in a bowl and mix well. Make up to two days in advance.

Meaty Red Beans and Rice

Ingredients

- 1 tablespoon olive oil
- 1 cup diced yellow onion
- 3/4 chopped red bell pepper
- 1 stalk celery, diced
- 2 cloves garlic, minced
- Kosher or sea salt to taste
- 1/4 teaspoon cayenne pepper
- 1/2 teaspoon freshly ground black pepper
- 2 teaspoons freshly snipped thyme
- 1 bay leaf
- 2 (15 ounce) cans dark red kidney beans
- 3 cups chicken broth (low sodium, fat free)
- 2 cups uncooked long grain brown rice
- SAUSAGE INGREDIENTS:
- 1 lb lean ground turkey or chicken, 93% works well
- 1/2 teaspoon garlic powder
- 1/2 teaspoon ground black pepper
- 1 teaspoon dried sage
- 1/2 teaspoon red pepper flakes
- 1/4 teaspoon cayenne pepper
- 1 teaspoon dried oregano

Preparation

1. For the sausage:
2. Place all the above sausage ingredients into a large mixing bowl and mix thoroughly until well blended. Make into small meatballs, about 1/2". Refrigerate while veggies are cooking.
3. For the beans:
4. In a large skillet, heat olive oil to medium-low, add onions, bell pepper and celery, sauté until tender, about 4 minutes. Add garlic and sauté one additional minute. Add sautéed onion, bell pepper, celery, garlic and remaining ingredients to the slow cooker, stir to combine.
5. Add sausage meatballs and stir gently, cover and cook on low 6-8 hours. Recommend 4-6 quart slow cooker.
6. For the rice:
7. Separately, cook brown rice according to the directions on package.
8. To serve:
9. Remove the bay leaf and serve sausage meatballs and beans over a bed of brown rice.

Chicken Stroganoff

Ingredients

- 6 boneless, skinless chicken breasts
- 1 can Amy's Cream of Mushroom Soup
- 16 oz. whole milk plain yogurt
- 2 Tablespoons dry, minced onion
- 2 MSG-free beef or chicken boullion cubes
- 1 large clove minced garlic OR 1 teaspoon garlic powder
- 16 oz. chopped, fresh mushrooms or your choice (we love baby bellas)
- 1/2 cup dry white wine
- freshly ground black pepper
- chopped fresh or dry parsley for garnish

Preparation

1. Put fresh or frozen, boneless-skinless chicken breasts in the bottom of a big crock pot. Mix remaining ingredients, except for the parsley, pour over chicken and cover. Cook on low for 6 to 7 hours. Salt to taste. Serve on noodles, potatoes, spaetzle dumplings or rice. Garnish with parsley. Delicious paired with a glass of pinot grigio.

BBQ Beef Sandwiches

Ingredients

- 1 (3 1/2-pound) eye-of-round roast, cut in half vertically
- 2 teaspoons salt, divided
- 2 garlic cloves, pressed
- 1 (10-ounce) can condensed beef broth
- 1 cup ketchup
- 1/2 cup firmly packed brown sugar $
- 1/2 cup lemon juice
- 3 tablespoons steak sauce
- 1 teaspoon coarse ground pepper
- 1 teaspoon Worcestershire sauce
- 12 Kaiser rolls or sandwich buns
- Dill pickle slices

Preparation

1. Sprinkle beef evenly with 1 teaspoon salt.
2. Stir together remaining 1 teaspoon salt, garlic, and next 7 ingredients. Pour half of mixture into a 5 1/2-quart slow cooker. Place beef in slow cooker, and pour remaining mixture over beef.
3. Cover and cook on HIGH 7 hours.
4. Shred beef in slow cooker with two forks. Serve in rolls or buns with dill pickle slices.

Buffalo Chicken Lettuce Wraps

Servings: 6 • Size: 1/2 cup chicken + veggies • Old Points: 3 pts • Points+: 3 pt

Calories: 147.7 • Fat: 0.1 g • Carb: 5.2 g • Fiber: 1.6 g • Protein: 24.9 g • Sugar: 1.7 g

Sodium: 879 mg

Ingredients

- 24 oz boneless skinless chicken breast
- 1 celery stalk
- 1/2 onion, diced
- 1 clove garlic
- 16 oz fat free low sodium chicken broth
- 1/2 cup hot cayenne pepper sauce (I used Frank's)
- For the wraps:
- 6 large lettuce leaves, Bibb or Iceberg
- 1 1/2 cups shredded carrots
- 2 large celery stalks, cut into 2 inch matchsticks

Preparation

1. In a crock pot, combine chicken, onions, celery stalk, garlic and broth (enough to cover your chicken, use water if the can of broth isn't enough). Cover and cook on high 4 hours.

Honey Sesame Chicken

Prep time: 10 mins

Cook time: 4+ hours

Ingredients

- 6 skinless chicken thighs, bone-in
- 1/2 an onion, finely chopped
- 2 cloves garlic, minced
- 1/2 cup honey
- 1/2 cup low-sodium soy sauce
- 4 tbs tomato puree/paste
- 2 tsp sesame oil
- 3 tsp cornflour/cornstarch
- 1/4 cup water
- 2 cups broccoli florets, chopped into bite sized peices + 1tsp sesame oil for frying
- Rice or quinoa, to serve
- Toasted sesame seeds, to serve

Preparation

1. Place the thighs in the bowl of a slow cooker.
2. Combine the onion, garlic, honey, soy sauce, tomato puree and oil in a bowl, and pour over the chicken. Cook on low for at least four hours, preferably six, turning occasionally to ensure the thighs cook evenly.
3. 20 mins before you want to serve, prepare the rice according to packet instructions, and remove the chicken from the slow cooker.

4. Combine the cornflour and water in a cup or small bowl to create a slurry, and add it to the remaining sauce in the slow cooker, turning the temperature up to high to allow the sauce to thicken. While it thickens up, shred the chicken with a fork and discard the bones.
5. Add the shredded chicken back to the thickening sauce, turning the mixture occasionally.
6. In a skillet or frypan, heat 1 tsp of sesame oil over a medium-high heat. Stir fry the broccoli pieces, until they turn a fresh rich green colour and their outsides look moist, but they're still fairly firm to bite (no mushy broccoli here, thanks!)
7. Lay the broccoli over the rice, and top with a good dollop of the chicken/sauce mixture, then sprinkle with sesame seeds. Couldn't be easier.

Rancher's Roast Beef

Ingredients

- 1, 2-3 lb beef chuck roast
- ½ tsp kosher salt
- 2 tbsp canola oil
- 1 (.4 oz) packet ranch dressing mix or 1 tbsp homemade ranch mix
- ½ C sliced pepperoncinis
- ¼ C pepperoncini juice
- 2 tbsp butter
- 2 C beef broth
- 1 tbsp corn starch
- ½ C sour cream

Preparation

1. Heat canola oil over med-high heat. Season roast with salt and sear in hot oil until golden brown.
2. Place roast in crock pot and sprinkle with dressing mix, pepperoncinis, pepperoncini juice, and dot with butter.
3. Cook in crock pot on LOW for 6-8 hours or HIGH for 3 ½ -4 or until the roast is fork-tender. Remove meat from pot and drain off cooking juices into a sauce pan, skimming the top for excess fat. Add 2 cups of beef broth to the juices and bring to a boil.
4. Mix 1 tbsp of corn starch with ¼ C of COLD water and slowly pour into the boiling broth mixture. Stir continuously until thickened and remove from heat. Stir in ½ cup of sour cream into the thickened broth and serve over the cooked meat.

Coconut Curry Chicken

Ingredients

- 2 lb boneless skinless chicken breasts or chicken thighs, cut into cubes
- 5 large carrots, peeled and diced
- 1 medium onion, peeled and quartered
- 2 cloves garlic, peeled
- 1 large bell pepper, seeded and chopped (I used a green pepper)
- 1 (5 oz) can tomato paste
- 1 (14 oz) can coconut milk
- 1 1/2 tsp salt
- 1 tbsp curry powder
- 1 tbsp garam masala
- 1 jalapeno, seeded and halved OR 1 tsp crushed red pepper flakes
- 2 tbsp water
- 1 1/2 tbsp cornstarch

Preparation

1. Grease your slow cooker with Pam. Place the chicken and carrots on the bottom of slow cooker.
2. Place the rest of the ingredients (except water and corn starch) in a food processor and process together until mixture is mostly smooth. •••If your food processor is too small to hold everything, process everything but the coconut milk. Transfer mixture to a medium bowl then mix in the coconut milk.
3. Pour the sauce over the chicken and carrots, mix well, then cover and cook on low for about 6 hours.

4. An hour or so before serving, mix cornstarch and water together in a small bowl until cornstarch is dissolved. Pour mixture into the slow cooker, stir to combine, and continue cooking for another hour.
5. ••This will thicken up the sauce. When the sauce is to your desired thickness, turn slow cooker to warm setting until ready to serve.
6. Serve over rice, with Naan, and garnish with cilantro.

Pulled Pork

prep time: 10 minutes

cook time: 8 hours

total time: 8 hours, 10 minutes

yield: serves about 8

serving size: 1 cup

Ingredients

- 3 onions, sliced
- 2 apples, peeled and cubed
- 1 bonelss pork shoulder
- 1 tbsp paprika
- 1/2 tbsp cumin
- 1/2 tbsp cinnamon
- salt to taste
- 1 tbsp honey
- 1 cup beef stock
- 1/2 cup apple cider vinegar
- fresh cilantro for garnish

Preparation

1. In a small bowl, combine spices (paprika, cumin, cinnamon) and salt. Rub the pork shoulder with the mixture.
2. Make a bed of onions and apples at the bottom of your slow-cooker, and place pork shoulder on it. Drizzle with honey. Pour beef stock and apple cider vinegar.
3. Cook on low for 8 hours.

4. When meat is cooked, transfer it to a plate (be careful, it will easily fall apart!) and shred it using two forks. Transfer onion and apple mixture to a colander and drain it. Keep about 1/3 of the liquid, or enough to moist the meat.
5. Combine meat, onion and apple mixture and add some liquid if necessary. Garnish with fresh cilantro.

Wine and Tomato Braised Chicken

Ingredients

- 4 slices bacon
- 1 large onion, thinly sliced
- 4 cloves garlic, minced
- 1 teaspoon dried thyme
- 1 teaspoon fennel seeds
- 1 teaspoon freshly ground pepper
- 1 bay leaf
- 1 cup dry white wine (see Tip)
- 1 28-ounce can whole tomatoes, with juice, coarsely chopped
- 1 teaspoon salt
- 10 bone-in chicken thighs (about 3 3/4 pounds), skin removed, trimmed
- 1/4 cup finely chopped fresh parsley

Preparation

1. Cook bacon in a large skillet over medium heat until crisp, about 4 minutes. Transfer to paper towels to drain. Crumble when cool.
2. Drain off all but 2 tablespoons fat from the pan. Add onion and cook over medium heat, stirring, until softened, 3 to 6 minutes. Add garlic, thyme, fennel seeds, pepper and bay leaf and cook, stirring, for 1 minute. Add wine, bring to a boil and boil for 2 minutes, scraping up any browned bits. Add tomatoes and their juice and salt; stir well.
3. Place chicken thighs in a 4-quart (or larger) slow cooker. Sprinkle the bacon over the chicken. Pour the tomato

mixture over the chicken. Cover and cook until the chicken is very tender, about 3 hours on High or 6 hours on Low. Remove the bay leaf. Serve sprinkled with parsley.
4. Variation: Turn 2 cups each of leftover chicken and sauce into Braised Chicken Gumbo. Heat 1 tablespoon extra-virgin olive oil in a large saucepan over medium heat. Add 1 diced medium red or green bell pepper and 2 tablespoons all-purpose flour and cook, stirring, until the pepper is beginning to soften and the flour is golden brown, about 2 minutes. Add 2 cups shredded chicken, 2 cups sauce, 2 cups reduced-sodium chicken broth, 1 cup sliced okra (fresh or frozen, thawed), 3/4 cup instant brown rice (see Tip) and 1/8-1/4 teaspoon cayenne pepper. Bring to a boil. Reduce the heat and simmer until the flavors meld and the okra is tender, about 10 minutes.

Hungarian Beef Goulash

Ingredients

- 2 pounds beef stew meat, (such as chuck), trimmed and cubed
- 2 teaspoons caraway seeds
- 1 1/2-2 tablespoons sweet or hot paprika, (or a mixture of the two), preferably Hungarian (see Ingredient Note)
- 1/4 teaspoon salt
- Freshly ground pepper, to taste
- 1 large or 2 medium onions, chopped
- 1 small red bell pepper, chopped
- 1 14-ounce can diced tomatoes
- 1 14-ounce can reduced-sodium beef broth
- 1 teaspoon Worcestershire sauce
- 3 cloves garlic, minced
- 2 bay leaves
- 1 tablespoon cornstarch mixed with 2 tablespoons water
- 2 tablespoons chopped fresh parsley

Preparation

1. Place beef in a 4-quart or larger slow cooker. Crush caraway seeds with the bottom of a saucepan. Transfer to a small bowl and stir in paprika, salt and pepper. Sprinkle the beef with the spice mixture and toss to coat well. Top with onion and bell pepper.
2. Combine tomatoes, broth, Worcestershire sauce and garlic in a medium saucepan; bring to a simmer. Pour over the beef and vegetables. Place bay leaves on top. Cover and cook

until the beef is very tender, 4 to 4 1/2 hours on high or 7 to 7 1/2 hours on low.
3. Discard the bay leaves; skim or blot any visible fat from the surface of the stew. Add the cornstarch mixture to the stew and cook on high, stirring 2 or 3 times, until slightly thickened, 10 to 15 minutes. Serve sprinkled with parsley.

Stuffed Peppers

Ingredients

- enough peppers to fit your crockpot. I have a 6qt oval Smart Pot, and six nestled perfectly in the stoneware
- 1 lb lean ground beef
- 1 cup cooked rice
- 1 can flavored tomatoes (I used fire roasted, Italian would work. If you don't have flavored, add ½ t italian seasoning)
- 1 t gluten free worcestershire sauce
- 2 T ketchup
- 1 t black pepper
- 1/3 cup water

Preparation

1. in a bowl, mix the ground beef and rice with all the stuff (except for the water and the peppers)
2. wash and clean out the peppers. Save the tops.
3. Stuff each pepper with a good amount of the ground beef and rice mixture
4. Nestle the peppers into your crock and put the little pepper tops back on.
5. Pour in 1/3 cup of water around the bases of the peppers
6. cook on low for 6-8 hours. I cooked these for exactly 8.

Turkey Osso Buco

Ingredients

- 1 teaspoon dried thyme
- 2 whole turkey legs (about 3 1/4 pounds total), cut at joints into drumsticks and thighs, skin removed
- 1 tablespoon olive oil
- 2 medium onions, coarsely chopped
- 2 medium carrots, peeled, chopped
- 2 celery stalks, chopped
- 6 garlic cloves, minced, divided
- 1/2 cup dry red wine
- 1 28-ounce can diced tomatoes in juice
- 1/4 cup chopped fresh Italian parsley
- 1 teaspoon grated lemon peel

Preparation

1. Rub thyme over turkey; sprinkle with salt and pepper. Transfer to 6-quart slow cooker. Heat oil in large nonstick skillet over medium-high heat. Add onions, carrots, and celery; sauté 8 minutes. Stir in 4 minced garlic cloves. Transfer vegetables to slow cooker. Add wine to skillet; boil until reduced by 1/3, about 1 minute. Pour wine and tomatoes with juice over turkey. Cover; cook on high until turkey is very tender and falls off bone, about 5 1/2 hours.
2. Mix parsley, peel, and remaining garlic in bowl for gremolata. Using slotted spoon, remove turkey from pot. Pull meat from bones; divide meat among 6 bowls. Season sauce with salt and pepper; spoon over turkey. Sprinkle with gremolata.

Moroccan Lamb
Ingredients

- 1 whole lemon, diced (do not peel)
- 1 teaspoon sugar
- 1/2 teaspoon kosher salt
- 2 whole lamb shanks
- Salt and freshly ground black pepper
- 2 teaspoons olive oil
- 1/2 large onion, diced
- 1 red bell pepper, diced
- 2 cloves garlic, minced
- 1 can diced tomatoes
- 1 1/2 cups water
- 1 cup canned garbanzo beans, rinsed and drained
- 1/2 cup whole olives, drained
- 2 cinnamon sticks
- 1 teaspoon kosher salt
- 1 teaspoon ground cumin
- 1 teaspoon ground coriander
- 1/4 cup golden raisins

Preparation

1. To make the quick-preserved lemon, combine diced lemon, sugar and salt. Mix well and let sit at room temperature while you continue with recipe.

2. Remove as much of the tough, silvery membrane from the lamb shanks as possible. Season all over with salt and pepper. Heat olive oil in frying pan and sear lamb shanks on all sides, about 7 minutes total. Remove lamb shanks and return pan to stove on medium-low heat. Add the onion, bell pepper and garlic. Saute for 2 minutes and then add to slow cooker. Pour the diced tomatoes, water, garbanzo beans, olives, cinnamon sticks, salt, cumin and coriander into the slow cooker and mix well. Add the lamb shanks and spoon some of the vegetable mixture over them. Turn slow cooker on high for 4 hours or low for 8 hours.
3. Halfway through cooking, stir in the raisins and half of thepreserved lemons. (Store the remaining preserved lemons in refrigeratorfor another use.)

Shrimp and Artichoke Barley Risotto

Ingredients

- 3 cups of water•
- 3 teaspoons Better than Bouillon Lobster Base•
- 1 cup chopped onion
- 3 cloves of garlic, minced
- 1 9oz package frozen artichoke hearts, thawed and quartered
- freshly ground black pepper, to taste
- 1 cup (200gm) pearl barley
- 1lb shrimp, peeled and deveined
- 2oz parmesan or pecorino romano cheese, grated
- 2 tsp grated lemon zest
- 4 oz baby spinach
- salt and pepper, to taste

Preparation

1. Bring 3 cups of water to a boil. Whisk in the lobster base and set aside.
2. In a nonstick skillet over medium-low heat, saute the onions until tender, about 5 minutes. Add the garlic and cook for 1 more minute, stirring. Transfer to the slow cooker and add the artichoke hearts, black pepper, and barley. Stir in the lobster broth. Cover and cook on high for 3 hours, or until barley is tender and the liquid is just about all absorbed.
3. About 15 minutes before serving, stir in the shrimp and grated cheese. Cover and continue to cook on high for another 10 minutes, or until shrimp are opaque. Add the lemon zest and fold in the baby spinach, stirring until it's

wilted. Season to taste with salt and pepper. Divide among serving bowls and serve immediately.

•In place of the lobster base and water, you can use 3 cups of seafood or chicken broth.

Cedar Plank Salmon

Ingredients

- 1 cedar plank
- 1 1/2 pound salmon fillet
- 1/2 teaspoon salt
- 1/4 teaspoon freshly ground black pepper
- 1 lemon, sliced
- 1 tablespoon grainy mustard
- 2 tablespoons maple syrup
- 1 tablespoon butter
- 1 teaspoon finely minced fresh parsley

Preparation

1. Cut plank to fit slow cooker. (If you need help, ask your handiest friend with a small hand saw.) Using tongs to hold the plank, char the plank for a couple minutes on both sides over an open flame. Soak plank for 1 hour or up to overnight.
2. Place plank inside slow cooker. Season salmon with salt and pepper on both sides and place on top of slow cooker. Scatter lemons on top of salmon. Cook on low for 2 hours.
3. Discard lemon. Slow-cooked salmon will always have some white protein on surface, which is perfectly fine.
4. In a microwave-safe bowl, combine the mustard, maple syrup and butter and melt. Pour over salmon. Garnish with parsley.

Loaded Baked Potatos

Ingredients

- 4 medium russet potatoes
- 2 tablespoons olive oil
- 10 ounces cremini mushrooms, trimmed and quartered
- 1 bunch broccoli, cut into small florets, stalks peeled and cut into 1/2-inch pieces
- Salt and pepper
- 1/4 to 1/2 cup vegetable or chicken broth, hot
- 2/3 cup low-fat plain yogurt, room temperature

Preparation

1. Wrap each potato in foil and place in a 5-to-6-quart slow cooker. Cover and cook on low until potatoes are tender, 8 hours.
2. In a large skillet, heat oil over medium-high. Add mushrooms and cook 2 minutes, then add broccoli and season with salt and pepper. Cook, stirring frequently, until broccoli is crisp-tender, 8 minutes.
3. Split potatoes, scoop out flesh, and transfer to a medium bowl, reserving skins. Add broth and yogurt to bowl, then season with salt and pepper and stir until combined; divide among potato skins. Top each stuffed potato with broccoli mixture.

Vegetarian Tamale Pie

Ingredients

- 1 med. onion, chopped
- 2 C. frozen soy burger crumbles
- 1 15-oz. can kidney beans, drained, rinsed
- 1 10-oz. can enchilada sauce
- 1 6.5-oz. pouch golden corn muffin and bread mix
- 1/3 C. milk
- 2 Tbs. butter or margarine, melted
- 1 egg
- 1/2 C. shredded Colby-Monterey Jack cheese blend
- 1 4.5-oz. can chopped green chiles, undrained
- 1/4 C. sour cream
- 4 med. green onions, chopped

Preparation

1. Spray 8-inch skillet with cooking spray. Add onion; cook over medium heat about 3 minutes, stirring occasionally until crisp-tender. In slow cooker, mix crumbles, onions, beans and enchilada sauce. In mediumbowl, stir corn bread mix, milk, butter and egg just until moistened. Stir in cheese and chiles. Spoon over mixture in slow cooker. Cover; cook on Low heat setting 4 hours 30 minutes to 5 hours 30 minutes or until toothpick inserted in center of corn bread comes out clean. Serve tamale pie with sour cream and green onions.

Barley Risotto with Fennel

Ingredients

- 2 teaspoons fennel seeds
- 1 large or 2 small fennel bulbs, cored and finely diced, plus 2 tablespoons chopped fronds
- 1 cup pearl barley, or short-grain brown rice
- 1 small carrot, finely chopped
- 1 large shallot, finely chopped
- 2 cloves garlic, minced
- 4 cups reduced-sodium chicken broth, or "no-chicken" broth
- 1-1 1/2 cups water, divided
- 1/3 cup dry white wine
- 2 cups frozen French-cut green beans
- 1/2 cup grated Parmesan cheese
- 1/3 cup pitted oil-cured black olives, coarsely chopped
- 1 tablespoon freshly grated lemon zest
- Freshly ground pepper, to taste

Preparation

1. Coat a 4-quart or larger slow cooker with cooking spray. Crush fennel seeds with the bottom of a saucepan. Combine the fennel seeds, diced fennel, barley (or rice), carrot, shallot and garlic in the slow cooker. Add broth, 1 cup water and wine, and stir to combine. Cover and cook until the barley (or rice) is tender, but pleasantly chewy, and the risotto is thick and creamy, 2 1/2 to 3 1/2 hours on high or low.
2. Shortly before serving, cook green beans according to package instructions and drain. Turn off the slow cooker.

Stir the green beans, Parmesan, olives, lemon zest and pepper into the risotto. If it seems dry, heat the remaining 1/2 cup water and stir it into the risotto. Serve sprinkled with the chopped fennel fronds.

Vegetarian Lasagna

Ingredients

- 1 large egg
- 1 15- to 16-ounce container part-skim ricotta
- 1 5-ounce package baby spinach, coarsely chopped
- 3 large or 4 small portobello mushroom caps, gills removed (see Tip), halved and thinly sliced
- 1 small zucchini, quartered lengthwise and thinly sliced
- 1 28-ounce can crushed tomatoes
- 1 28-ounce can diced tomatoes
- 3 cloves garlic, minced
- Pinch of crushed red pepper (optional)
- 15 whole-wheat lasagna noodles (about 12 ounces), uncooked
- 3 cups shredded part-skim mozzarella, divided

Preparation

1. Combine egg, ricotta, spinach, mushrooms and zucchini in a large bowl.
2. Combine crushed and diced tomatoes and their juice, garlic and crushed red pepper (if using) in a medium bowl.
3. Generously coat a 6-quart or larger slow cooker with cooking spray. Spread 1 1/2 cups of the tomato mixture in the slow cooker. Arrange 5 noodles over the sauce, overlapping them slightly and breaking into pieces to cover as much of the sauce as possible. Spread half of the ricotta-vegetable mixture over the noodles and firmly pat down, then spoon on 1 1/2 cups sauce and sprinkle with 1 cup mozzarella. Repeat the layering one more time, starting with noodles. Top with a third layer of noodles. Evenly spread the

remaining tomato sauce over the noodles. Set aside the remaining 1 cup mozzarella in the refrigerator.
4. Put the lid on the slow cooker and cook on High for 2 hours or on Low for 4 hours. Turn off the slow cooker, sprinkle the reserved mozzarella on the lasagna, cover and let stand for 10 minutes to melt the cheese.

Vegetable Curry

Ingredients

- 4 medium carrots, sliced
- 2 medium potatoes, cut into 1/2-inch cubes
- 1 15 ounce can garbanzo beans (chickpeas), rinsed and drained
- 8 ounces fresh green beans, cut into 1-inch pieces
- 1 cup coarsely chopped onion
- 3 cloves garlic, minced
- 2 tablespoons quick-cooking tapioca
- 2 teaspoons curry powder
- 1 teaspoon ground coriander
- 1/4 teaspoon crushed red pepper
- 1/4 teaspoon salt
- 1/8 teaspoon ground cinnamon
- 1 14 ounce can vegetable broth or chicken broth
- 1 14 1/2 ounce can diced tomatoes, undrained
- Hot cooked rice

Preparation

1. In a 3-1/2- to 5-quart slow cooker, combine carrots, potatoes, garbanzo beans, green beans, onion, garlic, tapioca, curry powder, coriander, crushed red pepper, salt, and cinnamon. Pour broth over all.
2. Cover and cook on low-heat setting for 7 to 9 hours or on high-heat setting for 3-1/2 to 4-1/2 hours.
3. Stir in undrained tomatoes. Cover; let stand for 5 minutes. Serve over hot cooked rice. Makes 4 servings.

Garlic Cauliflower Mashed "Potatoes"

Ingredients

- 1 head of cauliflower
- 3 cups water
- 4 large garlic cloves, peeled
- 1 tsp salt
- 1 bay leaf
- 1 Tbsp butter
- Milk (if needed)
- Salt and Pepper

Preparation

1. Cut the cauliflower into florets and place in the slow cooker.
2. Add in the water, garlic cloves, salt and bay leaf.
3. Cover and cook on HIGH for 2-3 hours or on LOW for 4-6 hours.
4. Remove the garlic cloves and bay leaf. Drain the water.
5. Add in the butter and let it melt.
6. Use a potato masher to mash the cauliflower or if you want to use an immersion blender to make it more creamy you can do that. If it needs milk add it in a tablespoon at a time.
7. Salt and pepper to taste. Serve with chives or green onions.
8. •you could totally make this recipe on the stove top too! Just bring the water to a boil, add in the cauliflower, garlic cloves, salt and bay leaf. Then cook over medium heat until the cauliflower is tender. Remove the garlic and bay leaf and drain the water. Add in the butter with the cauliflower and let it melt. Use a potato masher or even a mixer to mash the cauliflower to the desired consistency. If it needs milk, add one tablespoon at a time. Salt and pepper to taste and serve!

Ratatouille

Ingredients

- 1/4 cup olive oil
- 2 red onions, chopped
- 3 Yukon Gold potatoes, chopped
- 3 large garlic cloves, peeled and smashed
- 2 small eggplant, ends trimmed, cut into large chunks
- 3 small zucchini, ends trimmed, cut into large chunks
- 4 bell peppers (assorted colors), seeded, cut into large chunks
- 3 medium tomatoes, seeded, cut into medium chunks
- 4 portobello mushroom caps, stems removed, cut into large chunks
- 1/4 cup white wine
- 2 Tbsp fresh thyme leaves (or 1 Tbsp fresh oregano leaves)
- 3 Tbsp balsamic vinegar, or more to taste
- Kosher salt and fresh black pepper, to taste
- 2 Tbsp arrowroot or cornstarch

Preparation

1. In a large sauté pan or skillet, heat the oil over low heat, and add the onions, potatoes and garlic cloves. Cook, stirring occasionally, for 3-4 minutes, until the onions just begin to get translucent and the garlic hasn't begun to brown. Transfer the contents to a 6- or 7-quart slow cooker.
2. Add the eggplant, zucchini, bell peppers, tomatoes, mushrooms, wine and thyme leaves. Cook on LOW for 3-1/2 hours, stirring once during that time.
3. Turn the cooker to HIGH, and add the balsamic vinegar. Season with salt and pepper to taste.

4. Mix the arrowroot or cornstarch with 6 tablespoons of water, to make a slurry. Pour that into the slow cooker and stir. Cover, and cook for 15-20 minutes on HIGH. The liquid in the cooker will be slightly thickened (and it will thicken more if you let the ratatouille chill in the refrigerator).
5. Serve hot, at room temperature, or cold.

Squash Lasagna

Ingredients

- 1 package of regular whole wheat lasagna noodles (I've used the "no boil" kind in the slow cooker too and both that and regular noodles work, so use whatever you have on hand)
- 2 10-oz. packages of frozen pureed squash or 2 cups of fresh pureed squash•
- ½ teaspoon of dried rubbed sage
- 1 15-oz. container of part skim ricotta cheese
- ½ cup of milk
- ¼ cup of parmesan, grated
- ¼ – ½ cup of part skim mozzarella, shredded
- A few handfuls of spinach (optional)

Preparation

1. In a bowl, combine squash with sage. Add salt and pepper to taste. In another bowl, combine ricotta with milk and parmesan. Add salt and pepper to taste.
2. Coat the inside of a 5-6 quart slow cooker with non-stick spray. Place a layer of noodles at the bottom (you will have to break them to make them fit – don't worry about using little pieces to fill in crevices, it will come out just fine). Cover with half of the squash mixture, spreading it evenly. Place another layer of noodles on top, then a layer of spinach and half of the ricotta mixture. Repeat layers, ending with ricotta. Sprinkle mozzarella on top. Cover and cook on low for 3-4 hours (until noodles are tender).
3. • To use fresh squash, cut in half, remove seeds and roast in a 400°F oven for around 45 minutes or until soft. Let cool, then scoop out flesh and puree in blender or food processor.

Indian Chole

Ingredients

- 2 cups of chickpeas soaked overnight
- 3 cloves garlic, minced
- 1 large onion, minced
- 1 red bell pepper, minced
- 2 14 oz can of diced tomatoes
- 1-inch piece ginger, minced
- 1 14 oz can of coconut milk
- 1/2 tsp cayenne pepper
- 1 tsp coriander powder
- 1/2 tsp turmeric
- ½ tsp ground cardamom
- ¼ tsp ground cloves
- 1 tbsp vegetable oil
- 1 tsp garam masala
- 1.5 tsp mustard seeds
- 1/2 tsp salt

Preparation

1. Blend all the ingredients but chickpeas in a food processor or a blender until liquid. Wash and drain chickpeas, place them in a slow cooker, pour the blended mixture over and cook on low for 6-7 hours or on high for 4-5.
2. Make ahead: we usually make double or triple of this recipe, since we love it. Let it cool, and store chole in freezer-safe zip-lock bags in the freezer for up to 6 months.

Banana Brown Betty

Ingredients

- 1/3 cup pure maple syrup
- ¼ cup unsweetened almond milk
- ½ teaspoon ground cinnamon
- ¼ teaspoon ground ginger
- ¼ teaspoon ground nutmeg
- 1/8 teaspoon salt
- 6 cups cubed white bread (see Note)
- 4 ripe bananas, peeled and chopped
- 1/3 cup chopped toasted pecans
- 1/3 cup packed light brown sugar or granulated natural sugar
- 2 tablespoons brandy or rum or 1 teaspoon brandy or rum extract

Preparation

1. In a large bowl, combine the maple syrup, almond milk, cinnamon, ginger, nutmeg, and salt and mix well. Add the bread cubes and stir to coat.
2. In a separate bowl, combine the bananas, pecans, sugar, and brandy, stirring to mix.
3. Lightly oil the slow cooker insert or spray it with nonstick cooking spray. Spread half of the bread mixture in the bottom of the cooker, followed by half of the banana mixture. Repeat the layering, then cover and cook on High until firm, 1½ to 2 hours. Serve hot.

Note: For gluten-free, use a gluten-free bread.

Poached Pears with Caramel Sauce

Ingredients

- 1-1/2 cups brown sugar
- 1 Tbsp grated ginger root
- 2 Tbsp unsalted butter, cut into small pieces
- 4 firm, slightly underripe Bartlett or Bosc pears
- 1/8 tsp ground cinnamon, for garnish

Preparation

1. In a 4-quart slow cooker, stir together the sugar, ginger and butter.
2. Peel the pears with a vegetable peeler. Cut each pear in half lengthwise, and use a melon baller to remove the core. With a sharp paring knife, remove the stem and trim the bottom.
3. Gently toss the pears with the sugar mixture in the slow cooker, and layer them cut side down.
4. Set the cooker to HIGH, cover, and cook for 2 hours, until the pears are tender when pierced with a knife. (Open the cooker once during the cook time and gently spoon the sauce over the top pears.) Turn the cooker off, and with a slotted spoon, remove the pears to a bowl.
5. Pour the caramel sauce into a small sauce pan, and bring to a boil. Reduce the heat to low, to keep the sauce at a simmer. Shaking the pan fairly constantly, reduce the caramel sauce by one-third of its original volume (don't let the caramel get too dark, or it will have a burnt taste), 2-3 minutes.
6. Place 1-2 pear halves per person on individual plates. Spoon a bit of sauce over the pears, and sprinkle with cinnamon. Serve warm.

Clean Eating Brownies

Ingredients

- 1 cup whole wheat pastry flour
- ½ cup cocoa powder, unsweetened
- 1-1/2 teaspoon baking powder
- 3/4 cup apple sauce, unsweetened
- 2 medium, ripe bananas, mashed
- 1 cup honey
- 4 egg whites
- 6 ounces unsweetened Baker's Chocolate (6 squares)
- 1 tablespoon coconut oil
- 1/2 cup walnuts (optional)
- Olive oil in an oil sprayer

Preparation

1. Line the bottom of your slow cooker with parchment by placing the slow cooker liner on a piece of parchment, drawing a line around the base and cutting out. After inserting the liner, spray the entire inside with an oil sprayer.
2. In a large mixing bowl, blend the flour, cocoa powder and baking powder with a whisk.
3. In the microwave (microwave safe bowl), melt the Baker's chocolate for 2 minutes, and then in 30 second intervals, stirring between each one until the chocolate is melted. Stir the oil into the chocolate.
4. In a separate large mixing bowl, blend the apple sauce, mashed bananas, honey, egg whites, and melted chocolate.

5. Combine well with the whisk. Pour into slow cooker liner and cook for 4 hours. A knife inserted into the middle should pull out clean. If not, continue to cook without the lid for an additional 1/2 hour. To remove, run a knife around the edge of the liner and flip upside down onto a clean surface. The brownie should slide right out. Allow to cool. Slice and serve.

Pumpkin Bread

Prep time: 15 mins

Cook time: 3 hours

Total time: 3 hours 15 mins

Ingredients

- ½ cup of oil
- ½ cup of sugar
- ½ cup of packed brown sugar
- 2 eggs (beaten)
- 1 15oz can of pumpkin
- 1½ cup of flour (sifted)
- ¼ tsp. of salt
- ½ tsp. of cinnamon
- ½ tsp. of nutmeg
- 1 tsp. of baking soda

Preparation

1. Blend the oil and both of the sugars into a large bowl.
2. Then, stir in the beaten eggs and canned pumpkin. Add the remaining dry ingredients and mix thoroughly.
3. Pour the batter into a greased or oiled bread pan. (I used a canola oil spray that worked just fine.
4. Now add two cups of water to your crockpot and place the pan into a crock pot.
5. Cover the top of the crockpot with eight-ten paper towels. This is to trap condensation and keep the bread from becoming mushy.

6. Place the crock pot lid on top of the crockpot (I tried to make sure the paper towels were trapped around the lid so they didn't slip) and bake on high 2½ to 3 hours.

Chocolate Fudge
Ingredients

- 2-1/2 cups Chocolate Chips, [I used dark chocolate chips because of their health benefits. Ghirardelli is a good brand and works well with this recipe)
- 1/2 cup coconut milk, (canned, not in a carton)
- 1/4 cup coconut sugar, optional honey or maple syrup
- Dash of sea salt
- 2 tablespoons coconut oil
- 1 teaspoon pure vanilla extract

Preparation

1. Fudge is perfect for the slow cooker because it doesn't scorch or burn.
2. Add chocolate chips, coconut milk, coconut sugar, salt, and coconut oil, stir to combine. Next, cover and cook on low 2 hours without stirring. It's important that lid remain on during the 2 hours.
3. After 2 hours, turn the slow cooker off, uncover, and add vanilla. IMPORTANT; Do not stir fudge mixture at this point. Allow to cool to room temperature, or it reaches 110 degrees with a candy thermometer.
4. Once cooled, use a large spoon, stir vigorously for 5-10 minutes until it loses some the gloss.
5. Lightly oil an 8"x8" square pan. Pour fudge into pan, cover and refrigerate 4 hours or until firm. This fudge is very rich and meant to be eaten on occasion as a treat.

Note: Canned coconut milk can be found in the Asian or organic sections of most grocery stores.

Brown Rice Pudding

Ingredients

- 2/3 cup long grain brown rice (My favorite for this recipe is Lundberg Long Grain Brown Rice)
- 1 teaspoon cinnamon
- 1/4 cup unrefined sweetener (In this recipe we used coconut palm sugar. Other alternatives are sucanat and honey)
- 1 (13 1/2 ounce) can lite coconut milk
- 1 2/3 cup low-fat milk
- 2/3 cup raisins (optional)
- 1 teaspoon pure vanilla extract

Preparation

1. Add rice, cinnamon and sugar to the slow cooker, stir to combine. Add both milks, stir to combine, cover and cook on low 3-4 hours, or until rice is tender and desired thickness has been reached. Just before turning off the slow cooker, add vanilla and raisins, stir to combine, cover and allow to set about 10 minutes after the slow cooker has been turned off. Add additional cinnamon and raisins for garnish. Recommend 4-6 quart slow cooker.
2. Note: Our rice was cooked in 3 1/2 hours on low and was more on the creamy side and not overly thick. Slow cookers cook differently, so check the pudding after 3 hours for doneness.

Lightning Source UK Ltd.
Milton Keynes UK
UKHW021008070521
383312UK00014B/991